This book is dedicated to everyone v aroma of a flower, because perhaps for you, like me, there is something absolutely spectacular in capturing that true magic.

"**Creating is living doubly. The groping, anxious quest of a Proust, his meticulous collecting of flowers, of wallpapers, and of anxieties, signifies nothing else.**"

— Albert Camus, The Myth of Sisyphus and Other Essays

All Rights Reserved. No part of this publication may be reproduced in any form or by any means, including scanning, photocopying, or otherwise without prior written permission of the copyright holder.

Copyright © 2015 Elizabeth Ashley - The Secret Healer

In 2007, I lost everything. My job, my business, my dignity and I suspected losing my home wasn't far behind. It all happened, like a bolt from the blue, on December 17th. I had been working so hard, I'd hardly thought about Christmas and then suddenly the fates stole in and, quite simply, Christmas could not happen in our house. I bought a few small gifts for my children and I spoke to my family and friends who all agreed spending money on gifts at such a time was just daft and so, to all intents and purposes, I opted out of Christmas.

And it was great!

I walked round town and looked at people's faces; I saw nothing but worry. Worry they might not be able to get the toy they needed. Panic that auntie Flo, whom they hadn't seen since last Christmas might not like the talc they'd bought her (or worse they'd bought her the same last year, and forgotten!) But most of all, how on Earth were they going to pay for it all when the credit card statements come in?

Merry Christmas?

Not a single one of them looked like the dreamers the adverts were touting to wrench money from their cold and weary fingers.

And me? Well, I was free of it. I witnessed the Christmas Rat Race with an outsider's eyes...and being an outsider...made me smile larger than ever being *inside* of that panic had.

Well, blimey! It was like Christmas Interuptus for me! I was stopped in my tracks and I saw what I had been doing for years and promised myself that even when life was back on track, December certainly wouldn't look like that for *me* again.

I have to say, I have two sisters, Natasha and Angela. Both of them approach Christmas like a military operation, planning all year for the presents they will make and mine are simply not in their class! Tash's are beaded masterpieces that make you want to cry they are so beautiful and Ang's are incredibly witty and funny always with a clever little verse attached. I'm never going to be able to top her Christmas Pudding Vodka that nearly blew my head off one year, but I have acquired some pretty sterling tricks of the trade over the years! My pièce de resistance will always be my Victorian recipe Christmas pudding with enough brandy and Newcastle Brown Ale to floor an entire navy, but this year I have decided to raise my game. Look out bathrooms and bedrooms of my extended clan, Elizabeth Ashley has bottles of essential oil and she's not afraid to use them!!!

Some of these recipes have been new to me, some I have been using for almost thirty years in the family business. All are simple and easy to do.

Incidentally, I am aware not all people inhabiting our beautiful planet are Christians and I hope the word Christmas has not put you off reading this book. I have warmth and love for any religion that aims for peace, but sadly every other will lose out to a carol service at Christmas for me. That said, please take it as read that aromatherapy *transcends* religion. It is a healing art and should be used by anyone who wants to make someone happier or healthier. I'd like to think any of our different gods would smile on that endeavour.

Now…

I sat on the train this week and listened to two ladies discussing how appalled they were that Christmas had already lurked into the supermarket. I'd rather have hidden under the table than admitted to them that I'd started writing this gifts book all the way back in July! I've turned into one of *those* people….!

For this book, it is essential though, because making handmade perfumes, for example, takes time. Phil Collins was right when he said you can't hurry love but what he didn't tell you is you can't hurry a benzoin fixative either! A really fantastic fragrance takes time to settle and mature. If you want to create your own range of scents, you need to get started now!

With this book I wanted to create something different from those saturating the marketplace currently. Here, you won't find 25 recipes for one specific product, but rather the methods to make 50 different products and the know how to make them your own.

Pablo Picasso once said "Learn the rules like a pro, so you can break them like an artist." Well said that man! And I hope that is the spirit I have managed to capture in this book. At each stage, I'll show you how to make bath bombs, melts, and inks candles...etc. along with a couple of recipes, but a gifted therapist understands how to pour some of his/her own love and energy into the blend. This is what I want for you.

I hope that come January, when all the presents have been used up and the chocolates have been eaten, that you want to get the book out and make something different for yourself this time. Or maybe you want to take what you have learned into the outside world and put a more constructive application into action. It is very deliberate that the recipes are dirt simple. I'm hoping the creativity they inspire might channel a whole new way of healing for you. Whether that be aromatic play dough for special schools, scented inks to write notes to people locked in a separate world of dementia, or some respite at bath times for a carer perhaps.

To quote Jessie J, *it's not about the money, money money...we just want to make the world dance! Forget about the price tag.* You with me then...? Come on, I'll show you the rules. Then you can go smash them all to bits!

# Table of Contents

Chapter 1: Planning Christmas!...................................................13

Chapter 2 – The Secret Formula................................................24

    Mindfulness of Safety ...........................................................24

    Safety data ..............................................................................25

    Blending ..................................................................................28

    Dilutions .................................................................................29

    The Secret Ingredient ..........................................................30

Gifts for the Bathroom...............................................................41

    Melt and Pour Soap .............................................................41

    Making the Soap ..................................................................43

    Bath Bombs ..........................................................................45

    Bath Melts .............................................................................48

    Bath Salts ..............................................................................49

    Foot Bath ..............................................................................52

    Bath Tea Bags .......................................................................53

    Basic Scrub Recipe ...............................................................56

    Epsom Salts ..........................................................................58

The Beauty Counter ...................................................................61

    Body Lotions ........................................................................61

    Lotion bars ............................................................................63

    Lip Balm ................................................................................65

    Hand Cream .........................................................................67

    Cuticle Cream ......................................................................70

    Perfume .................................................................................70

    Pendants ...............................................................................81

The Living Room and Study......................................................83

Coasters with aroma pads ............................................................... 83
Room sprays .................................................................................. 84
Scented Ink .................................................................................... 88
Scented paper ................................................................................ 89
Christmas Evaporator Oils ........................................................... 92
The Bedroom ..................................................................................... 98
Drawer Liners ................................................................................ 98
Knicker Pouches .......................................................................... 100
Sleep Pillow Sachet ..................................................................... 101
Eye Masks ..................................................................................... 102
Candles ......................................................................................... 102
Scented Tea lights ....................................................................... 103
Wheat Bags .................................................................................. 105
The Playroom .................................................................................. 108
Play Dough ................................................................................... 108
Finger Paints ................................................................................ 109
Scented Pencils ............................................................................ 110
Room Plaques .............................................................................. 110
The Garden ...................................................................................... 113
Sunburn lotion ............................................................................ 113
Mosquito repellent ..................................................................... 113
Insect Repellent Garden Twine ................................................. 114
Insect Repellent Plant Markers ................................................. 115
Conclusion ....................................................................................... 116
About the Author ............................................................................ 118
Other Books by the Author ........................................................... 120
Disclaimer ........................................................................................ 123

# PART 1

# Preparing for Success

## Chapter 1: Planning Christmas!

Too exciting! Not the C word, actually. You can keep that, really. But the whole planning thing really turns me on! No-one loves an agenda more than I, and a list...ooo how I love a list but....

Here's the thing, even for the stalwart "let's wing it and see" if you don't do this bit carefully and precisely, your budget is going to bust, I promise you. Put a couple of hours of thought in here, before you click the eBay mouse and you will thank me for it later, I guarantee you!

### Who are the presents for?

Simple, straightforward, but you are going to need two lists. Who needs pressies, full stop? Then another of: who you are going to *make* gifts for.

Add your list up.

Now, are there any trends in that list? Lots of ladies for instance, lots of gardeners maybe?

Because the objective here is going to be to identify how we can make many permutations of different things on a theme.

Here are a couple of examples:

Heart shaped Rose and Geranium soap, body lotion, bath bomb and candles.

Gardeners' hand cream, soap, insect repellent string, insect repellent plant markers.

- By making a theme we only need to invest in one mould and limited oils that will keep help to keep costs to a minimum. Bases only cost a fraction of the price in comparison to those particular tools.
- This repetition on a cohesive theme also looks stunning when packaged together and makes thoughtful, well thought out gifts.
- Making one large batch of a mix is far simpler and will save you time and money.
- You get the very best economic use out of your oils rather than spending $10 on a bottle of oil you might only use 2 drops from!
- Imagine how delicious it will feel to stack one luxury product on top of another as you bathe, all of them adding to the same beautiful, simple fragrance. (Design houses will charge you way over $100 for that privilege)

**TIP 1: You might feel it is boring to make the same blends over and over, but the recipient of the gift will love you for it. Remember simplicity is elegance.**

*Packaging*
**Tip 2: Think about packaging first. Leaving it until the end will mean the costs quickly rack up.**

You can buy jars and bottles specifically for the purpose, but actually for someone giving products as gifts, that is money for old rope!

Go to your kitchen cupboard and see what jars you have. Jam jars, mustard pots, pickled chillies, mint sauce...they are all in great little pots. If you bought an empty jar, it would likely cost you very little less than one with the contents in! Same applies for vinegar bottles or lemon juice...

If you buy a pasta sauce, you will have a great big jar that you can decant several jars of mustard into and it will keep for just as long. Just be sure you label it! Don't feel your jars have to match but...

**IF YOU HAVE SEVERAL THAT HOLD THE SAME AMOUNT CALCULATING MEASURES WILL BE SIMPLER.**

*Work on Your Look*
In the perfumery business, marketing and packaging are everything. Most of the money you spend on a bottle of scent goes towards branding, those sensuous adverts and gorgeous bottles they use. That's not accidental because people shop

with their eyes. A brand should say everything about the person that made them.

Pop over to http://www.jamlabelizer.com and choose what labels work well for you. This will also have a bearing on which oils you decide to go with to because, unconsciously we associate colours with fragrances. For example, if you go for an orange label which is upbeat and funky that will jar with floral blends, because the person opening it is expecting a citrus blast. For me though, it is always going to be nostalgic, wistful and Roses so I'd be looking at pink labels and my blends probably give that away for me.

The beauty of life is we are all different, so celebrate that. There is no reason why you can't have a half-naked bloke rocking no more than a six pack and a Rudolf G-string if that's what floats your boat. Identifying a look that you like, will help you decide which oils will work best in your blends and also get that cohesive (cheaper to produce) theme we are aiming for.  Some of the label designs are free, others you have to pay $8 a year for, but you might feel spending that can take your gifts to a whole new level.

Incidentally, you can stick these on with glue, or you can buy one big A4 sticky label and cut them out.

## *Customise Your Jars*

If you think your jars shout "Mint Sauce" from the roof top, (and incidentally I promise you, they won't) you might want to change the way they look a bit. How about frosting them? Glass etching spray is about £3 /$5 and looks great all over the bottle, or you could use a stencil of a flower etc. for a really stunning look. You might want to consider using some glass paints if you are any good with a paintbrush too. Again, it's an investment of not more than a few pence to get really individual results.

A warning here though, I promised you a relaxing and creative time. If I tried this I would end up having to pay for a new pair of French windows after I had launched the pot across the living room in frustration. If painting gives you stress and depression...step away from customising jars! Frankly, my dears...life is too damn short!


## *Look in the house first*

The power of EBay, when it first started, was that everyone had some tat lying around that someone else could use as treasure. Let's turn that on its head and make that treasure our *own*. Before you hit the shops looking for fancy boxes do you have shoeboxes under the bed you can cover? Are there baskets lying about? What could you use to line the boxes? I, for one, am always buying tissue paper to stick onto Easter bonnets and then squirrelling away the rest only to be forgotten. What colours have you got stashed? Might that dictate the colours you need to use on your labels?

For me, the most romantic packaging will always be an old faded music score, for you it might be a piece of old French script. Done right, newspaper can look super cool. When I searched yesterday I found vintage newspapers from 99p, and you could get the whole batch of presents out of one paper, if you were careful. Same applies for cookery books and old herbals. Wrapping paper, cellophane....work it baby. Put in the brainpower and graft here to reap stunning results Think this bit out first, get the look and then come back to start thinking about recipes.

What about adornments? Can you bejazzle with lace, sequins, silk or dried flowers or beads. What's lying about that we can use? Best case scenario, we don't spend a penny on packaging. With thought and foresight, you can definitely achieve that. More, re-using and upcycling gets a high five from Mother Earth.

***Tips: Soap is best wrapped in tissue paper because it will absorb moisture better. Plastic / cellophane tends to make it sweat. Better still, don't wrap it at all.***

**Creams and lotions absolutely must be in glass or lined aluminium bottles or jars. Essential oils corrode plastic.**

**Bath salts should not be kept in jars that have metal fixings (kilner /mason jars, for instance) because the salt corrodes the metal. Plastic lids are better.**

### Storage

Take it from a seasoned pro...making loads of presents will drive you the wrong side of insane if you haven't thought about where you are going to store them until the big day. It needs to be dark and cool. A stacker box under the bed works well, as long as you don't put the top on. Let the products breathe or they will sweat.

Clear your space before you start. This makes for easy tidying and a whole less stress...not to mention irritating sarcasm from the rest of the house!

### Set Your Budget

Now, I know it's rude to discuss money, but we definitely need to now. Realistically, what *can* you afford to spend? Try to get past the "Well, nothing actually" initial response because we need to start somewhere.

Set the budget, and then work backwards.

If, say, we can afford $50 / £30 and we have 10 people to cater for, that gives us a unit price of $5 or £3 each. Can we do that? Cost each recipe as a batch and then work backwards and usually the answer will be yes, easily.

Be smart with your essential oil choices, stick to three or four and work out from there.

Your budget might have to go up a tad, but if you have thought out packaging first, the chances are, it won't have to, much.

### Work out your time
Read your recipes properly. How much time does a product need to rest before you can use it? Mostly it will be a maximum of overnight, perfumes need a month and scented paper takes a week. Have you left enough time to fit them in?

Don't try to do everything in one week. Do one mix a day, or even one each week. Most recipes only take about half an hour, if that. They are easy to build into your schedule and it will prevent that feeling of pressure that holiday preparations can bring.

### Cutting Corners
Ahem, did I really say that? Ssshhh, don't tell.

Of course, you can cut corners, and actually, maybe you *should* because that it how you are going to best learn the properties of your oils and ingredients. Don't follow my recipes word for word. Adapt them, mess with them and make them more cheaply.

Here's what you **don't** do!

**Don't mess with the ratios of the ingredients.** You need to leave those alone. If it says something is 70% of the recipe leave it that way or it will split, crumble, whatever.

Here's what you **can** do...

Rosewater, other floral waters and hydrolats can be supplemented with just water. That's fine. The properties won't be as strong, but you will have the essential oils to do the work, so cool...cut that corner to preserve your budget if you want to do so.

Carrier oils or macerations are delicious, sublime and frankly here...a bit of a luxury. Buy a big bottle of sunflower oil. It is great for the skin, has little scent and will work adequately well. Olive oil is great too, but you might find it a little heavy unless I have mentioned it in a recipe.

**Purchasing Tips:**
If you have set a theme you should be able to:

Buy one multi mould that you can use over and over. (Like this one for example: http://www.ebay.co.uk/itm/Flower-Silicone-Various-Shape-For-Chocolate-Cake-Mould-Ice-Cube-Soap-Mould-Mould-/321598509033?var=&hash=item4ae0c3cfe9 – you will get six soaps, bombs etc. in one go and that will save you a great deal of time.

There is nothing to stop you using an ice cube tray if you have one. It looks less fancy, but so what?!

Avoid overly small and fiddly moulds, but also avoid going too big. The deeper they are, the longer it takes for products to dry through properly and also, of course...the more it will cost you to make them. Silicon moulds are easy to use, but I have used ordinary muffin tins in the past too.

**Buy your mould first** and then measure its capacity. You will need to know how much it holds to calculate your measures.

**Do two checks:**

Fill **ONE** of the flower/cube/heart inserts with flour, pat it down then pour the contents into a scale to measure how much it held. **Note down the capacity**. It will be vital later.

Next, do the same with water and then pour into a measuring jug. (If they are small it might be easier to fill all the inserts, measure the volume and then divide by the number of inserts. Again: **note down the capacity.**

**So why are we doing this?**

We need to determine how many units a mix will make with *your* equipment.

If your mould holds 100g, then a 1kg mix will make ten bombs etc. , but if you have a smaller 75g one, the mix will yield 13 and a bit of wastage. (You might want to invest in an ice cube tray to use up the excess and make some extra gifts or use them up yourself.

Taking this into consideration each time will ensure you always have enough ingredients and will prevent costly wastage.

# Chapter 2 – The Secret Formula

**Mindfulness of Safety**

Boring, boring, boring...I know.

But, actually, it is not. Because this is how you start to understand the glory of what the oils do. Essential oils do not have side effects, but they *do* have many main effects, so we have to check that using one doesn't disturb something else in a person. Let me show you with a cooking analogy. Ludlow is the food centre of Britain and we have the most incredible butchers. Last week, I bought some of their famous sausages called Ludlow Sizzlers. To say they have chilli in them is an understatement!

I must admit I had kind of forgotten how potent a kick they had and I cooked and stirred them into some rice. Easy meal. Very proud.

It was delicious but every mouthful got harder. My whole body was heating up. My mouth was gasping for water. I couldn't really construct a sentence for fear of letting too much air onto my already on fire tongue; oxygen seemed like it may be a very bad plan!

But I got a "Yep it was nice, thank you" from the silent one and we washed up and should have forgotten it.

Then next morning I went to the loo...

You get the picture. The oils in the chilli weren't just about taste they triggered loads of physiological effects and every oil will do that.

Some will thin the blood. Others will raise blood pressure, some will lower it. There are some which are not great for people with diabetes and lethal for those with epilepsy. There is no need to be scared of them, you just need to be thorough.

Download your free copy of <u>The Complete Guide to Clinical Aromatherapy and The Essential Oils of The Physical Body,</u> then when you choose your oils, double check against it to ensure nothing will cause any difficulties.

Here are some good pointers:


**Safety data**
Essential oils are not suitable for everyone. The way they encourage the hormones in the systems to alter and can create damaging effects in some groups.

The main people to have concerns are:

1. Diabetes sufferers
2. Epilepsy patients
3. Pregnant women

4. Breast feeding women

## *Diabetes*

People with diabetes can safely use most essential oils with the exception of angelica oil. It is worth keeping essential oils containing high ketone content to a minimum especially when the diabetes symptoms are erratic. Oils high in ketones are:

- Peppermint - Mentha x piperita

- Rosemary ct camphor - Rosmarinus officinalis ct camphor

- Rosemary ct verbenone - Rosmarinus officinalis ct verbenone/camphor

- Sage (Spanish) - Salvia lavandulifolia

- Spearmint - Mentha spicata

- Spike Lavender - Lavandula latifolia

- Turmeric - Curcuma longa

- Valerian (Root) Valeriana officinalis

- Vetiver - Vetiveria zizanoides

Dill - (*Anethum graveolens*) and Fennel - (*Foeniculum vulgare*) however, are balancing to the pancreas and as such these are very helpful to suffers.

*Epilepsy*

Neuro-toxic oils, dangerous not only to sufferers of epilepsy but also some types of schizophrenia too, are: **Rosemary, Fennel, sage, eucalyptus, hyssop, camphor and spike Lavender (Lavandula latifolia)** these are best avoided by these sufferers

*Pregnant Women*

The many actions that essential oils have, make essential oils dangerous in pregnancy. **All essential oils should be avoided during the first 16 weeks**. Throughout the rest of the pregnancy **avoid *Angelica, Black Pepper Clove, Cypress, Eucalyptus, Ginger, Helichrysum, Marjoram, Myrrh - Nutmeg, Oregano, Peppermint, Roman Chamomile, Basil, Cassia, Cinnamon bark, Clary Sage, Lemongrass, Rosemary, Thyme, Vetiver, Wintergreen, White Fir.***

*Breastfeeding women*

The taste of essential oils oozes through into breast milk and so you may find it puts baby off feeding. There are some oils however which the breast feeding mum may find useful. Carrot Seed Oil enhances milk flow, Geranium soothes engorged breasts and Marigold heals cracked nipples. All others should be used with care.

If baby does stop feeding stop using oils for a day and see what happens.

## Blending

In that same book, there is also a section on blending. Read that section again so you can remind yourself of the importance of the Top, Middle and Base notes. You might also want to download the free blending chart again. You can find that at:

https://buildyourownreality.leadpages.co/oils-chart-please

Personally, I am an *OK* blender. I tend to blend therapeutically rather than by fragrance, but because of my synaesthesia, my blends turn out just higher than satisfactory verging on sweet/pleasant. There are some people who have a magical nose and can create stunning harmonies with oils and naturally they go on to be perfumers. I'd love *you* to give it a try.

You might find, for instance, that I have added an oil into a recipe that might have contra-indications for someone. Let's say Rosemary…it is great for nerve pain, but has issues for people with epilepsy. Go back to the *Complete Guide* and find another oil which has the same properties we used it for in the blend i.e invigorating, then try to substitute the same note, so ideally since you will be taking Rosemary out, and it is a middle note, you will be able to find another middle note with the same but safer properties.

It sounds complicated but…here's a trick. If you are reading on the Kindle use the button with three lines on and type "invigorating" into the "search for" function and it will bring them all up. Likewise if you are reading the book on your computer, click ctrl F and you will be able to flick through all my recommendations.

Use my free blending chart to always ensure you have a mix of Top, middle and base (or head, heart and base as they are called in perfumery). Experiment, learn grow...use my recipes as stepping stones. They most certainly are not the final word.

**Dilutions**
The same rules apply as always, maximum dilution for an adult is 3%, 2% for someone in a weakened or fragile state and 1% for children. Note though....the term MAXIMUM dilution. 3% is *a lot*. Very few of the recipes I make have that strong a dilution. **Less is always more**. It is cheaper, more effective and, actually, usually smells better too. You can always add more up to 3%, but consider it to be like salt in the potatoes...test it, then add more. You can't take it out once it is in.

## The Secret Ingredient

Using the term The Secret is a bit of a naughty play on words with Rhonda Byrne's book and film, because I want to talk to you about the **power of intention** and its fundamental place in making therapeutic products.

When I trained to be a therapist, mum always used to tell me to charge the cream with love and frankly, my ever so wise twenty six year old self sniggered inwardly, because I *really* didn't get it.

I'd come from a family where everything was done with love, really. Mum made people better, dad sold cars and cared about it and when he got home he grew vegetables, mended washing machines and renovated old furniture. Of course, you put love into it. That's what people do.

Now, of course, I know this was actually a very rare thing. A precious thing. And actually focusing your love on something you are making, is a *personal* and *powerful* thing. It is the difference between an aromatherapist and someone who puts a couple of drops of oil into a blend, stirs it, packages it, and waits for the profits to roll in. Most importantly, it is the difference between a good product and a truly magical one.

### *Healing Energies*

If you read <u>The Essential Oils of The Mind Body Spirit</u> I speak about the aura and chakras extensively. Whilst these are useful to a therapist if you are doing a massage, in honesty, you don't have access to these if you are making a bar of soap for someone! They become redundant, and so one might be forgiven for thinking that healing *cannot* take place. But that simply is not so, for healing energy does not come from the subtle energies, or even from within for that matter, we take it from the universe. It is *cosmic* energy and every one of us can tap into it, should we so desire.

Consider yourself to be like a radio transmitter. The message does not come from you, it merely uses you as a conduit. It comes through you and this is the same with healing. I use the sun as an anchor for my healing because it is very easy for me to imagine the power of its source. Other people use the moon or even just the sky. All are fine because the energy is *all around* us.

Close your eyes and imagine a ray of white light coming right down from the celestial body, piercing through your head. Let it come in through your crown chakra (a violet light above your head), pouring down through your body, energising every part of you, through to your hands and passing through your palms and fingertips into your product. .

Easy to write and actually, despite cynicism that might be overwhelming some of you right now, very easy to do...with a very small amount of practice.

The Secret just as Rhonda Byrne would tell you, is *believe* you can do it, because you can.

The more you practice and the more you work on raising your vibration through meditation, through just being happy...whatever it takes....the easier healing will flow and the more effective it will be.

Two things to consider then...*I* can't meditate well and the thought of a vegan diet leaves me...well laughing in hysterical panic frankly. The Gimli Son of Gloyn mantle, given to me by an ex-boss, is because I do disgruntled better than anyone and as for the language that comes out of my sewer mouth...

You'd go a long way to find someone less "saintly" than me...and I can charge a pot of cream well.

So can you.

And remember...even if your first impact is relatively small...it is better than 99% of the essential oil products out there, because so few people do it!!!

Love, intention, healing energy, whatever you choose to call it, it's the cheapest ingredient you are adding to your mix and yet the most valuable.

### Being Present in Your Presents

I hope we all sense the importance of concentrating our efforts on one thing at a time.

Noticing things.

Watching

*Appreciating.*

It is not just healing energy for the product we are making, but also for *ourselves*. This is such an immense weapon against stress in our lives and truly it is the key to happiness, I feel. Just *be*.

Be quiet.

Don't rush the stirring and bottling. Just concentrate your energy on your mixing. Worries and anxiety dissipate, if you give them chance to find their space to exit.

Breathe in these beautiful healing oils and perhaps pop on the song which I think sums up mixing a product every time I do it.

Whether your God is Yahweh, Buddha, Allah, the sentiment feels the same:

*Be still, for the power of the Lord*
*Is moving in this place;*

*He comes to cleanse and heal,*
*To minister His grace.*

Even the staunchest atheists and agnostics *must* be able to sense a higher calling from healing, even if they feel, as I do, that that energy and will lives within me. I have chosen a congregational version from Beverley Minster because I like to think of every one of us, many voices across the planet, working to the same healing melody.

Be Still: https://www.youtube.com/watch?v=Py9EDciaQ64

Please, don't for a second, lose sight of the marvel of how incredible it is that these little bottles of oil carry healing properties from the soil. What else *could* that be described as, unless magical?

You are a sorcerer, and that is the highest blessing. Acknowledge the miracle that is plant healing in your hands.

So then…. Are you ready?

Let's go destroy the kitchen!!!

# PART 2

# The Recipes

Potentially I am doing this a very strange way around, but to me it seems to make things easier for you to co-ordinate. These are the *master* recipes. You might decide to pick one of these to replicate over and over in your products. There are also some recipes attached to certain products to help you to see how to adapt certain ones and see how the ingredient ratios work. There is no rule about which you pick, the whole point is for you to be able to adapt and improve. **You can use any recipe for any product**. I am starting with recipes for people with certain conditions first, simply because these are the ones that seem to cause people to worry the most!

All blends are in this section are in a 100ml carrier, but that could just as easily be 100g of bath salt, 100ml lotion or 100g of soap.

X 1 = 1 drop,  X 2 = 2 drops, X 3 = 3 drops and so on....

### *Safe and Therapeutic Diabetes Blends*

In 100ml carrier (mixed to a maximum 2% dilution for an adult because this is a vulnerable group. My recipe is weak enough to be safe also for a child – 1%)

### *Relaxation*
Camomile Roman *(Anthemis nobilis)* x 1

Geranium *(Pelargonium graveolens)*  x 1

Juniper - *(Juniperus communis)* x 1

### Invigoration
Dill - *(Anethum graveolens)* x 1

Fennel - *(Foeniculum vulgare)* x 1

Cypress - *(Cupressus sempervirens)* x 1


### Safe and Therapeutic Epilepsy Blends
In 100ml carrier (mixed to a maximum 2% dilution for an adult because this is a vulnerable group. My recipe is weak enough to be safe also for a child – 1%)

### Relaxation
Rose - *(Rosa damascena)* x 1

Vetiver - *(Vetiveria zizanoides)* x 1

Geranium *(Pelargonium graveolens)* x 1


### Invigoration
Lemon Balm *(Melissa officinalis)* x 1

Bergamot - *(Citrus bergamia)* x 1

Camomile Roman *(Anthemis nobilis)* x 1


### Safe and Therapeutic Pregnancy Blends
In 100ml carrier (mixed to a maximum 2% dilution for an adult because this is a vulnerable group.) Please only use essential oils after 16 weeks of pregnancy though.

### *Relaxation*
Lavender - *(Lavandula angustifolia)* x 2

Camomile Roman *(Anthemis nobilis)* x 2

Geranium *(Pelargonium graveolens)* x 2

### *Invigoration*
Not advised. I'd rather keep mum and baby chilled!

### **Safe and Therapeutic Post Natal Blends**

### *Relaxation*
Rose - *(Rosa damascena)* x 1

Lavender - *(Lavandula angustifolia)* x 1

Clary Sage - *(Salvia sclarea)* x 1

### *Invigoration*
Celery Seed - *(Apium graveolens var. dulce)* x 1

Cypress - *(Cupressus sempervirens)* x 1

Geranium *(Pelargonium graveolens)* x 1

Tell mum that sometimes babies don't like the taste of essential oils in the breast milk and it can filter through from the blood stream. If baby does decide to be a bit finicky with feeding, stop use with oils to see if it makes a difference.

**Safe and Therapeutic Blend for Aches and Pains**
Lavender - *(Lavandula angustifolia)* x 1

Juniper - *(Juniperus communis)* x 1

Black Pepper - *(Piper nigrum)* x 1

Clary Sage - *(Salvia sclarea)* x 1


**Safe and Therapeutic Blend for Period Pain**
Rose - *(Rosa damascena)* x 1

Clary Sage - *(Salvia sclarea)* x

Geranium *(Pelargonium graveolens)* x 2


**Safe and Therapeutic Blend for Anxiety**
Valerian - *(Valeriana officinalis)* x 1

Vetiver - *(Vetiveria zizanoides)* x 1

Camomile Roman *(Anthemis nobilis)* x 1


**Safe and Therapeutic Blend for Gentle Relaxation**
Lavender - *(Lavandula angustifolia)* x 1

Mandarin - *(Citrus reticulata)* x 1

Camomile Roman *(Anthemis nobilis* x 1


**Safe and Therapeutic Blend for Anxiety**
Neroli - *(Citrus aurantium)* x 2

Valerian - *(Valeriana officinalis)* x 1

Geranium *(Pelargonium graveolens)* x 2


**Safe and Therapeutic Blend in hope of Happier Days**
Rose - *(Rosa damascena)* x 1

Neroli - *(Citrus aurantium)* x 1

Bergamot - *(Citrus bergamia)* x 1

# Gifts for the Bathroom

## Melt and Pour Soap

Melt and Pour Soap must be one of the very best gift cheats around! Mum and I first started making soap for The Apothecary about 20 years ago and it was the biggest fuss out. It would take hours up on hours, but the effects were beautiful. They still are, in fact. She still uses the same method we created all those years ago adding in so much carrier oil that the soap actually floats on the water!!!

She used laundry soap as the first ingredient and we had to grate it. The bars were a kilo each so your arm would ache and I can still smell the acrid scent of the base as I type.

All bow before the melt and pour soap. Easy, easy, EASY and *beautiful*, I might add! The glycerine ones are transparent and so you can add food colours to make shining gems, if you like, personally though I love the goat's milk and glycerine ones.

Glycerine is used in skin care because it draws moisture up from the deeper layers of the skin. It is smoothing and nourishing (*That aside don't use any soaps on your skins too often, and never on your face, they are simply too drying.*)

The secret is you buy the base, you melt it, add some essential oil, pour it into a mould and leave it to dry…

See? Told you it was a fab cheat!!!

Buy the **_Glycerine Soap Base_** off EBay, Amazon or any craft store. The base makes the same volume of soap in the end product, so if you buy a 500g block, that's how much soap you will end up with. There are plenty of vegetable glycerines around, if you look hard enough, so there is no need to miss out if you have animal product concerns. This soap base will cost you around £8/kg $16/kg

Also, purchase a **_pretty soap mould._** There are hundreds of these on the market now, hearts flowers, even willies, if you feel so disposed! (Please don't give that to grandma!) Truly, there is so much variety available, take your time to design around your mould first. You will likely come up with some brilliant themes. **Top tip:** Don't go too small, they become too fiddly to get out. Best to get a multi mould which will do about six at a time to make the job simple and quick…remember you need to be able to keep your soap hot and fluid so you need to be able to work quickly. This likely to cost you £5 / 410

You also need to buy some **_surgical spirits_**, which I understand you call **_rubbing alcohol_** in the States. This is important because it pulls all the air out of the soap and stops you getting bubbles in the soap. If you can get it in a spray, even better because all you are going to use it for is to "grease your tin" like you would when you are baking a cake. About £3 / $5

You will need **_essential oils_** to fragrance them and perhaps you might want to use some cosmetic glitter or dried flowers to make something really special. Good strong choices are: Geranium, Rose, Sandalwood, Sweet Orange, Lemon Verbena, Basil…but feel free to use any you like really!!!

Good children's choices for sleepy time are: Lavender, Camomile Roman, Violet Leaf , Vetiver , Valerian. Spend what you like here! We'll say another £5 / $8 but you will have oil left for other projects.

If you want to steal a trick from a Big Momma whose child does a little too much playing in the batch and not enough washing…Spiderman in the middle works well too, you have the right size mould!!!! (I got all the Avengers for £6 and used a large silicon muffin tray)

Take time to think about your gift list and plan your moulds – or stamps, these are lovely too – around them.

OK, when you have received your goodies you can make a start.

**Making the Soap**
- Cut the soap into small chunks and either prepare in the microwave or in a Bain Marie.
- If you do not have a Bain Marie, find a bowl that will fit happily and safely on top of one of your saucepans and fill the pan with boiling water. Place the soap into the

top dish and it will melt gently without coming into contact with the water.
- Stir occasionally with a wooden spoon to help it to melt more quickly.
- If you are preparing in the microwave, place into a heatproof jug and keep blitzing on high for 15 seconds, then stirring.
- Continue until all the soap is melted.
- Add your essential oils to the usual 3% for adults, and 1% for children. Add any glitters or dried flowers at this point if you want them to be combined into the main soap consistency
- Spray your mould liberally with alcohol to get a really lovely sleek finish.
- If you want a layer of Lavender seeds, or a rosebud sticking out of the top remember to put them into the mould at this point
- Check the soap is thoroughly hot and melted and pour into the moulds.
- Using a jug makes it easier to get the mix completely into the hole without any over spill. Clean any spills off the edges so the end product is beautifully neat.
- Leave to cool and dry.
- It will take about two hours but I recommend leaving overnight before you turn out the mould.

Soap gets better as it dries so potentially it makes sense to do this as one of your first Christmas jobs. It will, however keep in the freezer if you need somewhere to store it!

Don't forget to package prettily. Tissue paper is wonderful because it will keep it really, really dry.

## Bath Bombs

These are a fun addition to bath repertoire, and whilst I have to admit they are not my cup of tea, teenagers adore them. They are easy to make, look sensational, and again we can co-ordinate them with the rest of the ranges we are making for a sleek and sassy gift basket…and, of course all these cohesion of using the same ingredients and equipment will also keep your unit price per fantastic gift deliciously low.

For the main fizzing element we need to use a blend of 3 parts baking soda and 1 part citric acid, and these two ingredients should always make up at least 70% of your mix.

Your binding agent can be either water or oil and needs to constitute 10-20% of your mix. As ever, you can get creative here and use floral waters, more exotic carrier oils or butters. I find using a small amount of witch hazel in blend useful because the alcohol evaporates and dries the mix very quickly.

As usual, keep your essential oils content to 3%. Add some luxury with dried petals, clays or glitters but keep these to less than 5% of the mix so it does not dry out.

Mixing them is an art. Mix all your dry ingredients first then drizzle your binding agent in, very slowly, stirring all the time to prevent caking. If you can use a spray, it works even better. Simply mist the ingredients, so then it is very easy to mould them. All you need to do is pat them into a mould and leave them to dry overnight.

Package these in tissue paper or another packaging that will absorb any excess moisture away from the bomb. Silica gel pouches are useful if you are storing for a while.

Let's have a go then...These will make 1kg which is about 10 good size bombs.

## *Frankincense - and Camomile Roman Bath Bombs*
*(Good luck trying not sleep through the alarm after this one..!)*

- 600g (21 oz.) baking soda
- 200g (7oz) citric acid
- 75 ml (3 fl oz.) Frankincense - (Boswellia carterii) hydrolat
- 25 ml (1fl oz.) witch hazel
- 50g (2 oz.) Camomile (Anthemis nobilis) flowers

- Frankincense - (Boswellia carterii) x 20
- Camomile Roman (Anthemis nobilis) x 10
- Lavender - (Lavandula angustifolia) x 10

## *Lavender Loveliness Bath Bombs*
- 600g (21 oz.) baking soda
- 200g (7oz) citric acid
- 75 ml (3 fl oz.) Frankincense - (Boswellia carterii) hydrolat
- 25 ml (1fl oz.) witch hazel
- 50g (2 oz.) Camomile Roman (Anthemis nobilis) flowers
- Frankincense - (Boswellia carterii) x 20
- Camomile Roman (Anthemis nobilis) x 10
- Lavender - (Lavandula angustifolia) x 10

### *Aromatic Allure Bath Bombs*
- 600g (21 oz.) baking soda
- 200g (7oz) citric acid
- 50 ml (2 fl oz.) Rose - (Rosa damascena) hydrolat
- 25ml Shea Butter
- 25 ml (1fl oz.) witch hazel
- 50g (2 oz.) Dried Rose petals
- Geranium (Pelargonium graveolens) x 20
- Vetiver - (Vetiveria zizanoides) x 5
- Sweet Orange - (Citrus × sinensis) x 5
- Sandalwood (Santalum album) x 10

## Bath Melts

These are so pretty especially if you can co-ordinate them with your soaps to look very swish. They are just three simple ingredients. This will make about four small melts. Small flatter moulds work better for these. Perhaps a pretty flat flower? Feel free to add seeds, petals glitters etc. as usual to the liquid mix.

- 50ml cocoa butter
- 1tbs almond oil
- 10-15 drops essential oil

Gently melt the cocoa butter in a Bain Marie. Let the cocoa butter melt very slowly. (If it starts to boil it turns a nasty brown colour so watch it closely)

Give it a stir with a wooden spoon.

Add a tablespoon of almond oil and then your essential oils.

Pour into your moulds and leave to set for about three hours, but they are best left over night. Store in a cool dry place.

**Bath Salts**

I think bath salts might be my favourite thing to make! When you open the lid the fragrance of the oils explodes into the atmosphere and it is like heaven. They take seconds to make and cost virtually nothing but you can make them really beautiful.

My top tip for these is dried flowers! Gather up every petal from a fading flower you can find. I love rose petals, jasmine - geranium, violets and monarda but lavender and camomile are gorgeous too. Naturally, you can also add herbs and leaves to create more of a medicinal than a beauty slant. I tend to add 1 part flowers to four parts salt but it by no means an exact science. Let your creative juices flow... that's as much of a medicine as the gift you are creating.

There is probably only one rule, and that is keep your ingredients dry. If you are washing your Lavender seeds, do it the day before and leave them between two sheets of kitchen paper to soak up the moisture ready for assembly the next day.

Simply measure your salt into a jug, and add everything else in. Give it a very good stir to make sure everything is combined. You can add colours too if you like, for pretty stripes and designs. I find the colour pastes I use for cake decorating work best, because they are drier, but still combine well. Use the tiniest dip of the wrong end of a tea spoon and then add more if you need too.

TOP TIP: Make a bit extra. When you check on these the next day, the salt will have settled and so it looks rather a measly gift...half a jar of salt!

### *Relaxation Bath Salts*
- 100g 4 oz. Sea Salt
- 25 g 1 oz. dried Lavender flowers
- Lavender - *(Lavandula angustifolia)* x 5
- Camomile Roman *(Anthemis nobilis)* x 3
- Geranium *(Pelargonium graveolens)* x 1

### PMT Bath Salts

Let's be fair, if we are already hormonally irritated by life, it might be a good plan to leave flowers out of this one, so we don't get even more annoyed about cleaning the bath...because no other beggar is going to do it are they!!!

- 100g 4 oz. Sea Salt
- Rose - *(Rosa damascena)* x 1
- Geranium *(Pelargonium graveolens)* x 1
- Lavender - *(Lavandula angustifolia)* x 1

### Romance Bath Salts

- 100g 4 oz. Sea Salt
- Rose - *(Rosa damascena)* x 1
- Sandalwood *(Santalum album)* x 1
- Ylang Ylang *(Cananga odorata)* x 1

### *Indulgence Bath Salts*
- 100g (4 oz.) sea salt
- 25g (1oz) Rose petals and geranium flowers
- Rose - *(Rosa damascena)* x 1
- Neroli - *(Citrus aurantium)* x 1
- Sweet Orange - *(Citrus × sinensis)* x 1

### Foot Bath

This is a variation on a theme really. It's bath salts for your feet! I think these are a blissful gift for anyone who works on their feet all day. There are a couple of combinations and permutations and feel free to make them into sets with lotions and scrubs or…chuck all the oils in together!

Salts can be quite corrosive so either use a plastic lid, or pop them into bags and boxes rather than jars

### *Aching Feet*
- 100g (4oz) Sea Salt
- Lavender - *(Lavandula angustifolia)* x 5
- Geranium *(Pelargonium graveolens)* x 3
- Juniper - *(Juniperus communis)* x 1

### *Sweaty Feet*
- 100g (4oz) Sea Salt
- Clary Sage - (Salvia sclarea) x 1
- Peppermint x 1
- Patchouli x 1

### *Athlete's Foot*
- 100g (4oz) Sea Salt
- Tea tree *(Maleleuca alternifolia)* x 1
- Sweet Basil - *(Ocimum basilicum)* x 1
- Lemon - *(Citrus limonum)* x 1

### *Foot Refresher*
- *Paddling in the river on a summer's day!*
- 100g (4oz) Sea Salt
- Spikenard *(Nardostachys jatamansi)* x 1
- Spearmint *(Mentha spicata)* x 1
- Geranium *(Pelargonium graveolens)* x 1

### **Bath Tea Bags**

These are so simple, especially if you have been gathering your Lavender seeds and Rose petals from the garden through the year, but you can always purchase them for very few pennies. These are nice if you get a bit irritated with floating bits in the bath. The warm water runs through them opening the cells of the plant and they offer up all their gorgeous benefits into the water and the air.

Have a look out for **empty tea bags**. They are very cheap you can buy 100 for £1.40 / $3

The dry flower matter is ripe with benefits but they can smell a bit dusky and old so adding essential oils ramps up their healing properties and makes then nicer gifts. Making these means you can play with plants that don't necessary have essential oils too, like hibiscus for example, or ones that might be prohibitively expensive. A bag holds about 3g of herbs, so if you buy 100g of plant matter, expect to make about 30 bags give or take.

Why not make a lovely personalised tag and staple it onto the end of the string?

Make an assorted box for a fun and thoughtful gift.

A couple of recipes for you:

### *Sedation Soak*
- 50g (2oz) Yarrow (*Achille millefolium)* flowers
- 50g (2oz) Camomile Roman flowers
- 50g (2oz) Lavender seeds
- Lavender - (*Lavandula angustifolia*) x 5
- Camomile Roman (*Anthemis nobilis*) x 3

### *Summer Breeze*
- 50g (2oz) Jasmine flowers
- 50g (2oz) Honeysuckle flowers
- 50g (2oz) Rose petals
- Geranium (*Pelargonium graveolens*) x 5
- Jasmine - (*Jasminum officinale*) x 3
- Myrrh - (*Commiphora myrrha*) x 1

### *Body Scrub*

Exfoliation is the key to radiant and healthy skin. It sloughs off the old skin cells and brings newer, fresher ones to the surface. It also unblocks pores preventing spots and leaves the route out of the skin open for better detoxification. After all, the skin is the biggest excretory organ in the body.

Consider scrubs to be a bit like sand paper! We have very course ones for certain parts of the body where the skin is thickest, like the heels of the feet, and then we have Body

Polishes that are much lighter and gentle. These are designed to refine the skin.

As ever, there is very rarely a pair of scales in view when I make them because I tend to chuck in a little bit of this, a little bit of that but....

**Basic Scrub Recipe**
- ½ cup of salt
- ¼ cup of oil
- Between 10 - 15 drops of essential oil

Nice detoxifying ones that are kind to the skin are: Cypress – Juniper, Bergamot, basil

More astringent ones which work well in blends would be: Lemon Balm, Grapefruit, Black Pepper, Ginger. Don't use any more than one drop of these ones.

To make a ***polish***, why not substitute salt for brown sugar, oatmeal or wheat germ?

A couple of recipes then…

### Lovely Limbs Scrub
Stimulate circulation and tone up the lymphatic system.

Cypress - (*Cupressus sempervirens*) x 5

Grapefruit - (*Citrus paradisii*) x 1

Sandalwood (*Santalum album*) x 4


### Warming Rub
Benzoin *(Styrax benzoin)* x 1

Black Pepper - *(Piper nigrum)* x 1

Sweet Orange - (*Citrus × sinensis*) x 3

Geranium (*Pelargonium graveolens*) x 6


### Bring It On, Day! I'm Ready for Ya!
(You'll be able to take on the world after this one. Invigorating and stimulating, these ingredients are some of the world's happiest medicines. This is a blend for a serious up-day!

Grapefruit - *(Citrus paradisii)* x 2

Bergamot - *(Citrus bergamia)* x 3

Sweet Basil - (*Ocimum basilicum*) x 4

NB: Bergamot is phototoxic and so I wouldn't take the risk of using this on a very sunny day, despite the quantity being so small. If you did want to avoid the "blotchy skin" concerns you could invest in a bottle of Bergamot -FCF instead.

## Epsom Salts
1kg Epsom Salts £8 / $15

These are still bath salts, but with a bit more of a medicinal twist. Regular readers of my books will probably groan inwardly as Liz climbs onto her Magnesium soapbox, because I feel it is one of the most deleterious things facing our society today.

Most of the population is now magnesium deficient because naturally, magnesium is formed in fruit as it ripens on the branch. Nowadays, we pick fruit very early and it ripens on our windowsills after we have bought it from the supermarket. Magnesium then, does not have chance to form. Whilst it can still be found in nuts and some green vegetables it is a very really societal problem.

Scientists also suspect that the pandemic spread of Non Alcoholic Fatty Liver Disease may be attached to magnesium deficiency. On the very mildest scale it is attached to insomnia, anxiety, inability to concentrate and restlessness as well as health problems as diverse as incontinence and restless legs and even metabolic syndrome which leads to diabetes and heart disease.

We need more magnesium, people! One of the best ways to do this is with Epsom salts baths, because magnesium is actually best absorbed through the skin, and is found in Epsom salts. It is not an expensive product, but if you feel you want to "cut" some of the recipe with sea salt or rock salt to keep the price down…absolutely. Go ahead.

### *Insomnia Bath*
- 100g (4oz) Epsom Salts
- 2 tbs Bicarbonate of Soda
- Lavender - *(Lavandula angustifolia)* x 5
- Camomile Roman *(Anthemis nobilis)* x 5
- Valerian - *(Valeriana officinalis)* x 5

### *Restless Legs Bath*
- 100g (4oz) Epsom Salts
- 2 tbs Bicarbonate of Soda
- Lavender - *(Lavandula angustifolia)* x 5
- Clary Sage - *(Salvia sclarea)* x 5
- Geranium *(Pelargonium graveolens)* x 5

### Aching Muscles Bath
- 100g (4oz) Epsom Salts
- 2 tbs Bicarbonate of Soda
- Lavender - *(Lavandula angustifolia)* x 5
- Juniper - *(Juniperus communis)* x 5
- Geranium *(Pelargonium graveolens)* x 4
- Black Pepper - *(Piper nigrum)* x 1

### Anxiety Bath
- 100g (4oz) Epsom Salts
- 2 tbs Bicarbonate of Soda
- Geranium *(Pelargonium graveolens)* x 5
- Clary Sage - *(Salvia sclarea)* x 5
- Valerian - *(Valeriana officinalis)* x 5

## The Beauty Counter

My book: *50 Easy Essential Oil Recipes for Skin Care Products for Dry Skin* will teach you how to make moisturiser, night creams, toners etc. so they are not covered in this book. Clearly, though, they make über-fab pressies, so you might want to buy that book too, to add even more variety to your gifts.

## Body Lotions

If you are lazy (like me) you can buy lotion bases very simply and easily and then just mix your oils into them, adhering to the rule 3% dilution, unless it is for a child and then we reduce to 1%. If you want to have a crack at creating your own, here's how to do it.

As you will remember from school: oil and water will not mix. So to help them bind together we use an emulsifier called **emulsifying wax**. You may find these labelled as *cetearyl alcohol* and *polysorbate 60* or simply *Ewax*. You can find these easily on Amazon and EBay. This time our ratios are.

- 55% water base
- 35% oil
- 2% glycerine
- 2-5% Emulsifying wax (E/W)
- 3% Essential oils (E/O)

Take your E/W and place into a Bain Marie. Allow it to warm and melt in its own time over a medium heat.

Boil the kettle and measure out your boiling water or warmed hydrolats

Pour the meted E/W and water into a food processor, add the carrier oil and mix.

Watch your mixture. You want it well mixed, but not full of air otherwise it will sink when it cools. I find it easiest to pulse the blender.

If you are adding E/Os now, drop them in and give one more quick blitz to ensure they are blended.

Use a jug to pour into sterilised jars / bottles.

Do not put the tops on until they are completely cooled, otherwise you will have an outbreak of fungus on the top.

### *Sandalwood and Sweet Orange Body Lotion*
- Makes 500ml
- 175ml (7 fl oz.) water
- 100 ml (4 fl oz.) Sweet Orange Flower Water ( *Citrus × sinensis*)
- 175 ml (7 fl oz.) Evening Primrose Carrier Oil
- 10 ml (2 tsp) glycerine

- 25g (1 oz.) Emulsifying wax (E/W)
- Sandalwood (*Santalum album*) x 10
- Petitgrain - (*Citrus aurantium*) x 10
- Camomile Roman (*Anthemis nobilis*) x 3

## *Winter Warmer Body Lotion*
- Makes 500ml
- 175ml (7 fl oz.) water
- 100 ml (4 fl oz.) Sandalwood Hydrolat (*Santalum album*)
- 175 ml (7 fl oz.) Calendula Carrier Oil
- 10 ml (2 tsp) glycerine
- 25g (1 oz.) Emulsifying wax (E/W)
- Ginger - *(Zingiber officinale)* x 5
- Vetiver - *(Vetiveria zizanoides)* x 5
- Black Pepper - *(Piper nigrum)* x 3
- Myrrh - *(Commiphora myrrha)* x 2
- May Chang - (*Litsea cube*a) x 1

## Lotion bars

I love these as add-ons to your bottle of lotion; a gorgeously coordinated and classy gift. They look like soaps but they absorb into the skin when you rub them on. Again, we are looking to utilise our special moulds to get a really cohesive theme…and keep our unit cost low! Here we add in wheat germ oil to get a mega blast of vitamin E and to increase the healing potency of the oils. Coconut oil works well because it is solid at room temperature.

Here is your master recipe:

- 100g (4 oz.) Coconut Oil
- 100g (4 oz.) Shea butter
- 70g (2.5 oz.) Beeswax
- ½ tsp wheat germ oil
- 20 drops of essential oil

Melt your coconut oil, Shea butter and beeswax in a Bain Marie slowly and gently. When they are liquid turn the heat off the burner but leave the pan on the ring to keep warm.

Now squirt your moulds with rubbing alcohol (surgical spirits) to prevent them sticking.

Add your wheat germ and essential oils to the liquid, then pour into your moulds.

Leave to set over night.

## Lip Balm

In the biting winter, this is blissful relief from the Shropshire wind and rain. Package them into tubes or pots for a gift that your loved ones will adore you for.

- 15-20% beeswax
- 25-30% nut butter
- 45-50% oil

If you want the lip salve to be more rigid – like a stick- add more butter and wax. More oil will make it glossier. A word of warning though, the glossier it is the more often you will have to reapply. It won't stay on as long.

If you want to colour these, you could add some **Mica based colours**. To flavour them, you *can* use essential oils but **natural flavour oils** work better. For more subtle tastes why not use carriers or perhaps a bit of honey?

Very simply, melt your wax and butter together and then add in your oils and essential oils.

Stir gently to distribute them through the mix.

Decant into your pot or tube.

Leave to set overnight. Put tops on after about an hour.

I'll whip up some tasty ideas for you.

A 100ml mix will be ample for these. You only need teeny tiny pots.

### Rose hip and Blackcurrant Lip Balm
- 15-20g (1 tbs + 1tsp) beeswax
- 25-30g (1 oz.) Shea butter
- 20ml (1 tbs + 1tsp) Rosehip oil
- 30ml (1 fl oz.) almond oil
- 1 ml blackcurrant flavouring (add to taste)

### Mint and Honey Lip Tingle
- 15-20g (1tbs + 1tsp) beeswax
- 25-30g (1 oz.) Brazil nut butter
- 20ml (1tbs + 1tsp) apricot kernel oil
- 25ml (1fl oz.) olive oil
- 1 Tsp honey
- Peppermint essential oil x 1

NB: Please do not use this one for children as there are concerns about small children and peppermint e/o)

### Rose Lip Balm
- 15-20g (1 tbs + 1tsp) Beeswax
- 25-30g (1 oz) Cocoa butter

- 20ml (1 tbs + 1tsp) Apricot kernel oil
- 30ml (1 fl oz.) almond oil
- Rose - (*Rosa damascena*) x 1

## Hand Cream

So, now we are going to take the lotion base, add more emulsifying wax and make it thicker. Here we'll add skin healing oils to repair even the most battered of skins. Incidentally if you have someone in the family who has Raynaud's or who has permanently cold hands we can zip up their circulation here too.

Go luxury with Rose and Jasmine, practical for gardeners and woodworkers with a drop of Myrrh, or more clinical with some circulation boosters.

### Your master recipe:

- 50% water base
- 35% oil
- 2% glycerine
- 10% E/W
- 3% Essential oils (E/O)

Take your E/W and place into a Bain Marie. Allow it to warm and melt in its own time over a medium heat.

Boil the kettle and measure out your boiling water or warmed hydrolats.

Pour the meted E/W and water into a food processor, add the carrier oil and mix.

Watch your mixture. You want it well mixed, but not full of air otherwise it will sink when it cools. I find it easiest to pulse the blender.

If you are adding E/Os now, drop them in and give one more quick blitz to ensure they are blended.

Use a jug to pour into sterilised jars / bottles.

Do not put the tops on until they are completely cooled, otherwise you will have a mould outbreak.

### *Luxury Hand Cream*
### *100ml mix*

- 30ml water
- 20ml Rosewater
- 35ml Evening primrose oil
- 2% glycerine
- 10% E/W
- Geranium (*Pelargonium graveolens*) x 5
- Rose - (*Rosa damascena*) x 2

- Cedarwood Atlas- (*Cedrus atlantica*) x 5

## Gardeners Gratitude
- 30ml water
- 20ml Camomile Roman Hydrolat (*Anthemis nobilis*)
- 25ml Calendula oil
- 10ml jojoba oil
- 2% glycerine
- 10% E/W
- Myrrh - (*Commiphora myrrha*) x 5
- Galbanum - (*Ferula Galbaniflua*) x 1
- Petitgrain - (*Citrus aurantium*) x 5

## Circulatory Success – Bye Bye Cold Hands!
- 50ml Water
- 25ml Borage oil
- 10ml sea buckthorn oil
- 2% glycerine
- 10% E/W
- Geranium (*Pelargonium graveolens*) x 5
- Black Pepper - *(Piper nigrum)* x 1
- Ginger - (*Zingiber officinale*) x 5

## Cuticle Cream

This is the same principle as the <u>hand cream</u> really. Just make it a bit more "buttery" and put it into a smaller pot!!!

- 50ml Rosewater
- 25ml Rosehip oil
- 10g Cocoa butter
- 2% glycerine
- 10% E/W
- Myrrh - (*Commiphora myrrha*) x 1
- Neroli - (*Citrus aurantium*) x 1
- Vetiver - (*Vetiveria zizanoides*) x 1

## Perfume

What could be more exquisite than your own bespoke blended perfume? They are the epitome of refinement and luxury. Making perfume is not difficult to do, but it is time consuming and the ingredients are costly. That aside, how wonderful to wear a scent designed exclusively for you.

These directions are direct from the wisdom of Jill Bruce and her lovely shop. The Apothecary. I have to say I was very surprised she volunteered this "How –to" as readily as she has kept it a trade secret from even me for about two decades! I was very excitedly scribbling notes as she described the process.

Judging from her wry smile though, I suspect she knows you will seek out some of her perfume so you can buy from a master blender!

You will need to seek out **_Perfume Grade Alcohol._** It used to be that you needed a license to obtain this, but it is no longer the case and it can be easily found. If you wanted to make a cheaper version you could use vodka for this, but given the value and quality of essential oils it seems a shame, here, to compromise.

First you need to make your fixative. This is what holds the fragrances in place so they do not evaporate or change

For this we create a **_benzoin tincture._**

To do this add 1 tsp of benzoin resin (*Styrax benzoin*) and top up to 100ml. Over time the alcohol should dissolve the resin. This can take between a week to a month, so if it is not entirely disappeared, you may want to filter it to use.

## To make the Perfume

Your mix will be

- **2/3 Alcohol**
- **1/3 Fragrance**

Now, fragrance could mean essential oils, but here you can also afford to use fragrance oils which lend a whole new dimension to your scents.

Then you must add

- 2 tbs distilled water to each 300mls (10 ½ fl oz.) of alcohol

Store in dark glass bottles and shake every day for a week. After a week, then it is time to add the benzoin tincture as a fixative. The amounts of tincture you add depend on the strength of perfume you are trying to achieve.

*Your Tincture Ratios*
100mls of **perfume**

**Add 4tsp tincture** to 100mls of the alcohol/ oils mix

100mls **Eau de Cologne**

Add **10 tsp of tincture** and **50mls of distilled water** to 100 mls of the alcohol/oils mix

100 mls **of Eau de Toilette**

Add **15tsp of tincture** to **100 mls of distilled water** and 100mls of the alcohol/oils mix

Then comes the waiting game. You must leave them for a month to mature which gives the fragrances time to mingle and mature.

So, that all looks very easy, doesn't it? Of course, the skill is not in the process but in the practice of getting "the nose" right...ascertaining how the oils mingle and meld to make that complete accord of fragrances. I can give you some help here, but the expertise will always come by your own hand.

**Fragrance notes**

Whether an oil has a top, middle or base perfume note depends on what we call its volatility, that is: **how fast it evaporates.**

This tends to depend on its consistency. It makes sense that you would expect a thick gloopy oil to take longer to evaporate than a light thin one. Because of this, these oils have much deeper scents. They tend to be more soporific and sultry too.

Then, the faster they evaporate, the lighter and sharper the scent and we call those middle and top notes. When you speak in perfumery terms, rather than just blending terms we call:

- the top note - the head note
- the middle note - the heart note
- the base note - is the same!

A blend must have some of each note to make it resonate exactly. In effect when the perfumer gets it right, the chord- or, in fact, note...chimes beautifully.

You can download my blending chart which will help you a great deal.

It helps, I think to understand some of the fragrance families and how they work together.

The first family is called:

**Fougère,** which means fernlike.

Actually the translation helps us a bit because if you imagine walking through a forest on an autumn day, the fragrance of the russet bracken is a good comparison, I think.

It is a warm, woody and spicy fragrance. In fact the best scent you can imagine is oak moss, a really rich deep green scent, because all fougère perfumes need to have a base note of either oak moss or coumarin. Coumarin comes from the Tonka bean (*Dipteryx odorata)* and is very highly prized having a kind of deep vanilla fragrance.

The top note would usually be some kind of citrus or lavender with middle perfume notes blended to make each fougère fragrance different to the next.

Fougère fragrances can be sub classified again to include

**Fougère fresh** which would usually have herby oils mixed into give a lovely light fresh perfume.

**Fougère ambery** tend to have fragrances such as heliotrope to make them warm and comforting. These fragrances tend to feel like they are enveloping you. They are much softer aromas, a little reminiscent of vanilla and have a slightly powdery scent to them.

**Fougère woody** are exactly as you would imagine, Sandalwood, Vetiver and cedarwood; lovely woody scents.

**Fougère florals** are perhaps the most complex blends using lovely bright scents such as Sweet Orange blossom to harmonise with the woody-spiciness of the base notes. All **good Fougères have a rosy note at their heart** which could just as easily come from a plant such as the Geranium as from Rose - itself.

In more recent years, very popular fougère fragrances have been designed for men - the most well-known of these is Davidoff's Cool Water.

**Chypres** scents date back to when the crusaders brought labdanum (*Cistus ladanifer*) back from the east and the rich heady balsamic scent became a very popular base to perfumes. Chypres rely on a harmony between citrus aromas and woods. Another oil that is often used as a base note in these blends is patchouli (*Pogostemon cablin*).

Top notes tend to be Bergamot, Sweet Orange or Lemon and they have often have a floral middle note, so Rose or Jasmine - for example and then have perhaps a Sandalwood base note.

These fragrances tend to be your headier, "dressy" perfumes for the evening and because of the leaning to the large number of base note fragrances it will not evaporate quickly, lending itself to a perfume that you can rely on to last all evening.

**Green perfumes,** in a way, describe themselves. It can be frustrating that there are so few words to describe scents but there are very few truly green fragrances - pine needles, freshly cut grass, and cucumber.

These clever fragrances use herbs and leaves to bring that lovely clean fresh aroma.

**Florals** again need no explanation really. They could be single note perfumes like the lavender of rose perfumes or lily of the valley, for example, or they could be our blends of different flowers. Again in top, middle and base perfume notes.

**Orientals** are made with the most unguent of the oils. Tree saps like Frankincense and Myrrh, for example. These are very heady and will, of course, be the longest lasting of all the perfumes.

Some years ago oakmoss was deemed to be a sensitizing agent and so now we only use to a maximum dilution of 0.1% because sometimes it can irritate the skin.

Here are some examples of blends you might like to emulate. These mixes will make 300ml of alcohol/oils mix.

### Fougère Woody

200ml Alcohol

100ml E/os comprised of

Head notes

- 20mls Bergamot - *(Citrus bergamia)*
- 10mls Lemon *(Citrus limonum)*
- 5 mls Lemon Verbena *(Aloysia citrodora)*
- 5 mls Ginger - *(Zingiber officinale)*

Heart Notes:

- 10 mls Rose Otto - *(Rosa damascena)*
- 25mls Rose Geranium *(Pelargonium graveolens)*
- 15mls Palma Rosa *(Cymbopogon martini)*

Base Notes

- Oakmoss resin *(Evernia Prunastri )* x 10 drops
- Tonka *Bean (Dipteryx odorata)* x 10 drops
- Vetiver - *(Vetiveria zizanoides)* x 15 ml

**Fougère Fresh**

200ml Alcohol

100ml E/os comprised of

Head notes

- 15 ml Lavender - (*Lavandula angustifolia*)
- 15 ml Sweet Basil - (*Ocimum basilicum*)
- 5 ml Lemon Balm (*Melissa officinalis*)
- 10ml lemon verbena (*Aloisa citrodora*)

Heart Notes

- 25 ml Geranium (*Pelargonium graveolens*)
- 15 mls Petitgrain - (*Citrus aurantium*)

Base Notes

- Oakmoss (*Evernia punastri*) x 10 drops
- 10 ml Sandalwood (*Santalum album*)


**Chypres**

Head Notes

- 10ml Lemon - (*Citrus limonum*)

Heart Notes

- 20ml Petitgrain - *(Citrus aurantium)*
- 5 ml Neroli - *(Citrus aurantium)*

Base Notes

- 20ml Cedarwood Atlas- *(Cedrus atlantica)*
- 20 ml Patchouli – *(Pogostemon cablin)*
- 25 ml Sandalwood *(Santalum album)*

## *Floral*
## Head Notes

- 3ml May Chang - *(Litsea cubeba)*
- 2 ml Black Pepper - *(Piper nigrum)*
- 5 ml lemon – *(Citrus limonum)*

Heart Notes

- 5 ml Rose - *(Rosa damascena)*
- 20 ml Palma rosa *(Cymbopogon martini)*
- 5 ml Jasmine - *(Jasminum officinale)*
- 10 ml Tagetes *(Tagetes minuta)*
- 15 ml Ylang ylang *(Cananga odorata)*

Base Notes

- 25 ml Myrrh - *(Commiphora myrrha)*
- 10ml Cedarwood Atlas- *(Cedrus atlantica)*

*Labelling perfume*

Correct labelling is to detail the % of alcohol in the final mix so

- Perfume is 66%
- EDC is 57%
- EDT 50%

You should also list the active chemicals. That means if you don't want to give away the recipe you can list as the main chemical constituents

E.g. neral, geraniol etc. You can find these by searching "chemical constituents" of your chosen essential oil.

## Pendants

Aromapendants make really beautiful gifts and there is something very Zen about the process of them. If you are not familiar these are pendants made of very porous clay so when you put essential oils on them, when you wear them, they diffuse all through the day.

They are ace because unlike wearing perfume, you can actually use these to diffuse your medicine. In my book *The Aromatherapy Bronchitis Treatment* for instance, we created a blend of eucalyptus, ravensara and lavender to relax the patient and open the airways to make it easier for them to breathe.

So we are going to use any air dry clay. Usually you can get it in terracotta or white, so decide which will be easiest for you to wear.

Roll and cut out shapes, or make small beads.

If you are making a disc pendant, using stamps can give you really great designs. Personally I use the cutters I have in the drawer for making sugar paste flowers and leaves for cakes but you could be a whole lot more experimental.

Use a large needle or punch to make a hole large enough to thread your string or thong through

Leave to dry

The clay then becomes very porous and will hold your essential oils

Put one drop of oil on each bead or shape. Just in case of staining, do the back of each one.

Paint them up if you like!

Thread on and wear your medicine in style!!!

# The Living Room and Study

## Coasters with aroma pads

Are you a scrap booker? Do you have a flair with a pair of scissors or do you just like to see your kids squirm with dodgy pictures you have found of them? You'll love these. They are so easy and yet they great fun to give as stocking fillers.

In all seriousness, these are a clever addition to a stressed out student's bedroom. The idea is essential oils are activated by heat when they put their cup of tea onto them (C'mon! I'm English, you don't really expect me to write coffee there do you?)

You might also think about making a romantic one for by the bed in the morning? You know who you are creating for. Get imaginative.

We use ***diffuser pad refills*** for the oils. These cost about $3 £2 for a pack of six.

- Use the pad as a template and draw round it to cut out a circle in your picture, then also one the same size of card.
- Now assemble and glue together:
- Card on the bottom, then diffuser pad, then photo on the top.
- Put a couple of drops onto the side of the pad so they soak through the fibres and diffuse with the heat.

Ideas:

- **Relaxation**: Lavender - (*Lavandula angustifolia*) or Geranium *(Pelargonium graveolens)*
- **Seduction**: Ylang Ylang (*Cananga odorata*)
- **Dynamism**: Sweet Basil - (*Ocimum basilicum*)
- **Concentration**: Vetiver - (*Vetiveria zizanoides*)

Why not give your loved one a 1ml vial of each essential oil they might use? They can adapt the coaster to their mood.

## Room sprays

Synthetic room sprays improve the fragrance of a room, masking cooking smells and teenage room stench, but an *aromatherapy* room spray is something unique and enigmatic. Spraying tiny molecules of essential oil into a space diffuses them so the olfactory system can pick them up efficiently and continuously. But an essential oil is *more* than just a scent. It is hundreds of thousands of molecules capable of affecting the mood and disposition of the people inhaling them. Use the oils to aid concentration, to reduce stress and to bring about a happy party buzz.

Again we have an "oils and water don't mix" issue here, and so to help them to break up and dissipate more easily we are mixing in a tiny wee dram of alcohol. This also becomes helpful if you want to scent your curtains or sofa because it alleviates that delicious oily stain that an aromatherapy room spray might normally leave.

For this gift, you will need to think about your blending more deeply than for others. Firstly the fragrance is a standalone thing here, we are not particularly looking for anything else from that, apart from perhaps some emotional influences.

More specifically your blending will influence how your product performs. The citrusy, fresh top notes will unfold first, opening out to the heart note and then in time the dry down will allow the base note to come through.

Can you see how that is very different to a plug in thingy that just emits a lotus blossom or lavender scent into the room? This is a living thing, it morphs and changes.

So how can we use that cleverly?

Think about walking into a room, what would you want to happen?

1. You kick off your shoes, sit down, talk about your day and unload then vegetate in front of the TV. (We could go an uplifting "I'm home, tell me about your day mandarin top note. A camomile heart note unwind then a sedative benzoin to anchor it at the base)
2. Student walks into an exam room, terrified. Sits at his desk and stares bleakly at the paper. (How about an

empowering "Let's Do This" Sweet Basil top note, a hypnotic Clary Sage to help him access his revision memories more easily and then a deeply sedative Vetiver that improves concentration?

3. Friday night and wifey is a bit sick of playing second fiddle to the PlayStation; we'll go top note tuberose tingle (can't imagine what caused that strange stirring in the loins sensation...how very odd), then an exotic cardamom Come-on and finally a damiana dive on the bed!

See? Let the oils tell their own story....

How you package these are going to be up to you and this is very much going to affect your unit spend. The term to put into the search engine is "atomiser", otherwise you will get the little spray bottles that you mist plants with!

If you look for second hand ones of these you can get some real beauties. Incidentally, if you do come across any other old perfume bottles, vintage fragrances (with or without any scent in them) fetch serious pennies. Buy them, whack them onto EBay/ Etsy and you could make anywhere up to $100.

If you do go for a second hand atomiser be aware that, on the ones that have a puffball squirter, the rubber decays very quickly and often these no longer work.

In this case, because the quantity of essential oil is so diluted plastic spray bottles work well, and can be picked up for about 60p / $1 apiece. If you want to go very chic and tiny, you can also get atomiser pens that hold about 8ml each. The unit cost of the container isn't going to be that different, but the actual quantity of mix will be so much less, *that* will help keep costs down. The downside of these is they are very awkward to label because they are very slim and fiddly.

Again, here, sort out your packaging first, because if you need to buy in packs of four from a supplier, or perhaps you need to go for a different colour glass or even capacity, this could affect the entirety of your product.

### *Basic Room Spray Recipe*
- 300ml distilled water
- ½ tsp vodka
- Up to 9 ml essential oil - which in real money is about 180 drops!

What a waste! See what it smells like with 30 and work up from there!

TOP TIP: Use more drops of top note and less of base notes because by their very nature their fragrance is heavier.

Mix, shake, shake, and shake. The more you agitate the solution, the smaller the molecules will break down. This leads to more effective spraying.

**Scented Ink**
We live in a world where the written word is now king, but very few of us actually use a pen, let alone a fountain pen.

And yet...

How beautiful to get a handwritten note on scented stationary, written with a fragranced ink; so romantic and wistful.

This is a gorgeous way to make wedding invitations, Christmas cards and thank you notes, something very personal and unique. And they take seconds to make! Blends do work, but actually single notes are better for this. Geranium is my favourite, but Sandalwood, Lavender and Patchouli all work well. Top notes are not spectacular because they don't last very well and might evaporate from the paper before your recipient has time to enjoy them, despite the alcohol fixative!

- Buy a normal bottle of "Fountain Pen Ink".
- Place 1 tsp of vodka or alcohol into a glass jug. (If you use plastic it leeches into the jug...mine had to take on a permanent and rather disconcerting shade of baby blue for me to have found that out!)

- Add 20 drops of your chosen oil and then pour the ink on top of the mix.
- Stir thoroughly.
- Wash your ink jar ready for relabelling with your own pretty design.
- Decant the mix back into the jar and bottle any excess for your own use.

## Scented paper

It would take a very clever perfumer to make a blend of ink or paper that would complement each other, I think. Simply because the time elapses on the paper and in the liquid will be different. For that reason then, echo the same usage on the paper as you used for the ink. Lavender paper, Lavender ink, Geranium paper, Geranium ink and so on and so forth....

As ever we have a fear of oil staining her and the solution is to use blotting paper.

We use one small bookmark of blotter to each notelet we want to fragrance. It works better to do several at one time.

Use **3 drops of your chosen oil** on blotting paper and then fold it so there is no oil on the outside which could contaminate your pretty notelets.

Then put one bookmark into each card and then each card into its envelope.

Put the whole pile into a zip lock plastic bag for a week.

This will give the oils time to evaporate and get trapped on the fibres of the paper.

I would store these in their bag and probably give the blotting paper as part of the gift too, since it will help to preserve the enigmatic memory in the gift.

A couple of recipes for those of you who are not using ink. You can be more adventurous then, I think. Remember to consider your note dry down, top, middle base note. Since we are going for three drops *total* on each blotter, just one drop of each is adequate.

## **Cinnamon Christmas Cards**
One drop each of:

- T- Lemon *(Citrus limonum)*
- M- Cinnamon *(Cinnamomum cassia)*
- B- Myrrh - *(Commiphora myrrha)*

## **Frankincense Dream**
This is a must, I think, for those beautiful images of the nativity or the magi coming across the desert.

Frankincense is an extraordinary oil because, although in perfumery it is used as a base note, the way it unfolds means it also resonates as a top note. This is very helpful here, because it means we can squeeze Myrrh into the blend!!!This is a beautifully exotic blend that smells like the temple incenses of long ago.

One drop each of:

- T- Frankincense - - *(Boswellia carterii)*
- M- Cinnamon - *(Cinnamomum cassia)*
- B- Myrrh - *(Commiphora myrrha)*


### *Party Invitations*
Having a New Year bash? Let's go a bit more upbeat then.

One drop each of:

- T- Mandarin - *(Citrus reticulata)*
- M - Dill - *(Anethum graveolens)*
- B - Cedarwood Atlas- *(Cedrus atlantica)*


### *Looking to Pull!*
That's a separate one in a different bag then! How about a mysterious message of promise.

One drop each of:

- T – Lemongrass - *(Cymbopogon citratus)*
- M - Rose - *(Rosa damascena)*
- B – Labdanum – *(Cistus landifer)*

*Serious seduction!*

## Christmas Evaporator Oils

So, if the Christmas faery fluttered down from the top branch and offered us just one wish at 4pm on Christmas afternoon, what would we wish for? That the two sisters would stop bickering for just one day? For just one year, that that beautiful mellow haziness of the adverts might perhaps find its way into your living room? Or just to capture the fragrance of Christmas without a real tree! Evaporator oils are my secret weapon. I simply drop a couple of drips into the inconspicuous loaf tin on top of my wood burner and let the oils do their work. Their subtle medicine influences and affects the mood of everyone around me and calmness reigns...or that's the theory anyway!

Yours need not be as primitive as my loaf tin, these blends are great for candle evaporators and diffusers too. You might also want to use these blends when we get to the candles section.

I make these in 5ml bottles that I have emptied through the year, but you could just as easily do one drop of each straight into warm water for an immediate hit. Small bottles of different blends make a lovely gift for everyone, but especially those who have yet to be convinced of the power of the oils.

## Stir Up Sunday

My favourite day of the year is Stir Up Sunday when we pour buckets of booze and oodles of love (or is it the other way round, I forget!) into my great big stacker box to make all my Christmas Puds! Delia Smith says leave the fruit to soak overnight, but she is an amateur in comparison to me....for *three* days the house reeks of alcohol and spice. My kitchen is an utterly dreadful place to be!

But then, when all the steaming is over...the fragrance leaves and does not return until we turn on the box for the Queen's speech. That seems such a shame, so I like to recreate it as often as I can. This ties in the freshness of the tree and has a lovely sweet undertone with the Geranium and Myrrh.

- Sweet Orange - *(Citrus × sinensis)* x 20
- Lemon – *(Citrus limonum)* x 20
- Cinnamon - *(Cinnamomum cassia)* x 10
- Nutmeg *(Myristica fragrans)* x 10
- Juniper - *(Juniperus communis)* x 15
- Silver Fir – *(Abies alba)* x 15
- Geranium *(Pelargonium graveolens)* x 10
- Myrrh - *(Commiphora myrrha)* x 5

### Christmas Eve Tranquillity

My mum is a pagan and my husband is an atheist. There are few things they agree on, mother-in-law and son, but they are united in their exasperation of my deeply profound love of Christmas Carols. 4pm Christmas Eve, Carols for Kings is always accompanied by the resins of the magi.

In Ayurveda, Vetiver - (Vetiveria zizanoides) is called the oil of tranquillity and has a very strong smell in its own right, but as a weak note, I find it reminiscent of the hay from the manger

- Frankincense - (*Boswellia carterii*) x 40
- Myrrh - (*Commiphora myrrha*) x 15
- Camomile Roman (*Anthemis nobilis*) x 20
- Clary Sage - (*Salvia sclarea*) x 20
- Vetiver - (*Vetiveria zizanoides*) x 5

*Peace, perfect peace.*

If you listen carefully, you might even hear angels singing.


### Lingering Lunchtime

This is designed to be the antidote to "Let's get this over before they kill each other". Calm, friendly, loving....

- Mandarin - (*Citrus reticulata*) x 40
- Myrtle (*Myrtus communis*) x 30
- Camomile Roman (*Anthemis nobilis*) x 40

### *Mellow Mealtimes*
This one is a pricey one, but it is so silky smooth!

- Mimosa Absolute (*Acacia dealbata*) x 20
- Mandarin - (*Citrus reticulata*) x 40
- Galbanum - (*Ferula Galbaniflua*) x 30
- Vanilla absolute (*Vanilla planifolia*) x 10


### *Too Much Sugar Tranquilliser*
If yours is anything like my house, you might want to make a litre of this one! Worse than sugar "Turn that gizmo off!" You know the face and the foot stamp! The lemon verbena and Cypress are included to neutralise the positive ions off the electro-gadgetry.

- Lavender - (*Lavandula angustifolia*) x 20
- Camomile Roman (*Anthemis nobilis*) x 20
- Lemon Verbena (*Aloysia citrodora*) x 5
- Cypress - (*Cupressus sempervirens*) x 5
- Geranium (*Pelargonium graveolens*) x 40
- Valerian - (*Valeriana officinalis*) x 10

Oh by the way...there'll be a bonus with this one! You'll probably find they sleep!

### *Fir Tree Forgery*
If you want Scandinavia in your living room, without all the hoovering, essential oils are the perfect plan.

- Lemon (*Citrus limonum*) x 5
- Black Pepper - (*Piper nigrum*) x 5
- Juniper - (*Juniperus communis*) x 20
- Cypress - (*Cupressus sempervirens*) x 20
- Silver Fir (*Abies alba*) x 20
- Pine (*Pinus sylvestris*) x 20
- Cedarwood Atlas- (*Cedrus atlantica*) x 10


### *New Year's Resolution*
Willpower, motivation, encouragement. Come on New Year...Let's see what you've got!

- Sweet Basil - (*Ocimum basilicum*) x 40
- Neroli - (*Citrus aurantium*) x 20
- Sandalwood (*Santalum album*) x 40


Oh and if poor Uncle Bernard shows signs if having too many snifters of the barmaids apron, with his hands everywhere...We just know he's either going to get a slap or a pull something rather unfortunate...Marjoram, ladies. A drop of marjoram! That should dampen his ardour...but watch out...everyone else's in the room might start to wane too! And that's a neat little segue into the next chapter...matters of the bedroom.

## The Bedroom

In my Sweet Basil book, I talk about Ezulie Freda, the voudou Loa, or Goddess, of love. She and I have become friendlier recently, which is quite a shock to me frankly. Ezulie Freda loves pretty things, flirtation and perfumes. I have always been the scruffiest of creatures and not really had a very feminine disposition. Over the past few weeks that has changed and I have found I quite like being a bit more girlie. I feel more organised somehow, better put together, if that makes sense and I think that would be a lovely sense to give someone.

Here are some of the fripperies I have been experimenting with:

## Drawer Liners

These are lovely, and feel like such a nostalgic throwback to the past. You can buy them in shops but they seem to have a very powdery and synthetic fragrance, I have found.

We will use the same process as making the scented paper but this time we roll the paper around the blotters.

You can use wrapping paper for this, but I have found cotton and handmade papers seem to take the fragrance best. Don't use wallpaper. It is too thick for the oils to permeate very well.

It will take about 10 small strips of blotter to one piece of paper.

Use 3 drops of your chosen oil on blotting paper and then fold it so there is no oil on the outside which could contaminate your liner.

Lay your liner flat and then place one of the strips along the edge, and start to roll the paper. As you go, keep slotting in pieces of blotter into the roll.

If you are making more than one liner, keep rolling subsequent papers around the first so you have one big roll.

Secure the roll with a soft ribbon to prevent marking on the paper.

I use a bin liner to put my roll into.

Sticky tape round tightly so the oils are enclosed and trapped.

Find somewhere to leave safely for a week to ten days (Top of the wardrobe works well I've found!) This will give the oils time to evaporate and get trapped on the fibres of the paper.

Again, perhaps give the blotting paper as part of the gift too, since it will help to preserve the enigmatic memory in the paper and they slot beautifully between pretty knickers top fragrance them even more!

## Knicker Pouches

Vetiver - (Vetiveria zizanoides) gained fame and fortune when it came to Europe because Indian silks had been wrapped with Vetiver root tucked insides of the bales, to deter bugs and insects on its journey to the West.

Suddenly every lady in Paris wanted Vetiver pouches to scent their drawers. Exotic, seductive and moth free! It is possible to get "Vetiver Powder" fairly easily on the internet but because we are using wadding inside of these tiny pillows it is simple to use essential oil instead without the worry of marking.

I find these are prettiest if grouped in threes and tied in a stack with a ribbon. Choose three complementing fabrics for a lovely nostalgic feel.

*For each sachet*

- Cut two squares of fabric 14 cm on each side.
- On three sides hem together, wrong side of the fabric inwards, with a 1cm seam allowance
- Cut 5 pieces of 2oz wadding 12 cm round
- Either fragrance the middle three pieces of wadding with 5 drops of Vetiver oil or place Vetiver powder between the second and thirds layers of wadding.
- Gently push the sachets into their casing and hand stitch closed turning the hemming inwards.

Obviously, you need not use Vetiver, if you don't want to. Lavender, roses, camomile...whatever you choose will be beautiful.

Stack three cushions and secure with a ribbon or string and perhaps a pretty label.

**Sleep Pillow Sachet**
This is a variation on a theme really, because it is exactly the same thing as the knicker pouches but bigger, and designed to help insomniacs. Lavender is soothing and we are also going to add dried catnip leaves and flowers. It is almost hypnotic. Catnip is gorgeous and, of course, many people have it growing ion their garden. Cut the leaves and flowers close to the root and hang up for three or four days to dry. Cut up with scissors of pop into the food processor to really whizz it into tiny pieces and release loads of oil. Again, there is a lovely essential oil of catnip too.

Raise your fabric measurements to 35cm sq.

You will need to up your total wadding to about 3mtres. Again use herbs or oils between the layers.

A nice way to make this one slightly different is to cut a panel out of the fabric and lay tulle under. Perhaps a heart, a star or even cut out your friend's name, maybe? This is looks really effective if you put the herbs just beneath it because you can see them but also smell them better too.

## Eye Masks

Another variation on the theme; simply cut out the mask shape, instead. Will you go black satin and tuberose / ylang ylang /Sandalwood or floral and Lavender, Camomile or Geranium ...depends why you want the light out really, doesn't it?!

## Candles

These are also in my *Complete Guide* but they make such pretty gifts, I just had to add them in.

Simply choose uplifting oils, relaxing, stimulating or whatever effect you are looking for, to make your candle.

The easiest way is with a sheet of beeswax which you can buy from most craft shops or direct from a beekeeper. (EBay quite often lists them too.) The sheets come in rectangles and you can get 4 candles from each one.

- Cut the rectangle in half vertically and then cut each section diagonally to create two triangles.
- Smear some essential oil down the vertical edge of your triangle. Let it dry for a few moments then take a piece of cotton string to make a wick. Lay it along the same

vertical side then crease a small line of the beeswax against the wick to hook it into place.
- Roll the beeswax snugly around the wick. Wind it as tightly as you can against the string. Trim the wick to length.

Some people prefer to put the essential oil directly onto the wick but as it burns you lose the freshness of the scent that way.

For a gift though, I think it needs a little extra *something* something...why not add a little bee embellishment? (Search buttons, cabochon and bee embellishments for a quirky twist that completely reflects you...or even better *them*!) The wax is so soft you will be able to push it right in.


**Scented Tea lights**
This is the perfect cheat, so inevitably it is the one I always do! It is using plain old tea lights (plain white wax in a round foil container) and we are simply going to add some essential oil to their mix. If you are familiar with the stifling fragrance of synthetic candles, this subtle, mood enhancing product is absolute luxury. Essential oil candles sell for about $40 each, but you can make yours for pence.

The only difficult thing is controlling the wicks so....

Have some cocktail sticks at the ready!!

You say skillet, I say frying pan...Find the heaviest one you have, and ideally it will be the oldest and most battered you have!

With the stove burner turned *off*....

Fill your pan with as many candles as you can get in.

Pull all of your wicks up and very carefully lay cocktail sticks across the candle, either side of the wick to support it. You can even push it over to one side to prevent it from falling between them, if you are nervous.

When you are happy everything is secure, turn on the heat, very low.

The wax slowly turn to liquid but it is easier to control the wicks if you don't let it completely melt all the way through.

When you are happy the wax is warm enough, turn off the heat and add about 5 drops of oil to each candle. (Clearly you could also use a blend like the ones we made for the evaporator oils, and add 5drops of that.)

Leave the pan where it is for the candles to set. This will ensure you get a nice clean sheen to them.

For these...it's all in the packaging! Will you add to a hamper or package 6 in a box with a ribbon. Either way, they are guaranteed to be a hit!

**Wheat Bags**

I am a bit of a hot water bottle junkie. The first nuance of glum and I am a-cuddling. So I never quite understood the fuss about wheat bags until I had a bad neck. Then I really got it! If you make these right, you can twist and turn them around limbs or cosset poorly period tums and basically milk any illness you have for all it is worth!

They are very easy to make, cost virtually nothing and can be customised to be something very beautiful.

First tip: It doesn't have to be wheat inside. In fact, I like uncooked rice better. Here are some other ideas:

- Barley
- Beans
- Buckwheat hulls
- Cherry pits
- Feed corn
- Flax seed

- Oatmeal

Second tip: How about adding a little *je ne sais quoi* to the blend? You could add dry matter such as:

- Camomile flowers
- Cinnamon
- Geranium flowers
- Ginger
- Ground cloves
- Lavender
- Mint
- Nutmeg
- Rose petals
- Rosemary

And of course, you can add any essential oils into the pot pourri too, whether that be single notes of blends. If you are adding pot pourri, I would mix it the night before and let the scents diffuse through the smaller plant matter before mixing with the wheat etc. which is heavier for it to fragrance. You will get a more even mix then.

It works nicely to make the wheat bag and then make a little detachable case for it to go into that you can throw in the washer. If you co-ordinate with your loved ones furnishings this becomes a sweet little accessory in the bedroom.

- Cut your two pieces of cotton fabric, 28 cm x 15 cm (10 ½ " x 5 ½ ")
- Turn your fabric face inwards and sew up three sides (wrong side out) with a 0.5cm hem allowance. Then sew ¾ of the way along the forth edge. Leave a space open wide enough to put in a funnel
- This size bag will use about 500g of wheat or rice.
- Fill the bag and then neatly stitch the opening closed.
- Tie on a pretty label with the instructions:

*"Place in microwave with a small cup of water. Heat for two minutes on medium power."*

You might also want to add…

*"Keep a close eye during the heating for smoking"* because I have set mine on fire before now and my goodness the house stunk for days!

# The Playroom

## Play Dough

I love play dough. I don't love what it does to the carpet, but I do love play dough.

Homemade is lovely, because here we can use the oils to lift wee one's moods, access memories or even calm them during play. Here, they truly will be little sorcerer's apprentices!

The dough is simple to make. Go easy on the food dye. Less is definitely prettier!

- In a saucepan, mix together 1 cup flour, 1/2 cup salt, 2 tsp cream of tartar (or alum).
- Mix them together well then turn burner on to medium heat.
- Mix a couple of drops of food colouring and 1 tbs cooking oil into 1 cup water
- Mix the concoction into your dry ingredients and stir while it is cooking.
- Bring the dough together and ball, remove from heat. Turn onto the counter and knead.
- Add 10-15 drops essential oil AFTER the cooking process.
- Use your finger to draw a face in the dough and pour the essential oils into the holes!!!
- Knead it all together and then store in a big plastic container.

- **Happy oils**: Sweet Orange, mandarin, Lemon Balm, lemon verbena, Geranium, (especially for autistic children. Geranium seems to touch them in a way, I haven't seen other oils manage to do)
- **Oils for grief and sadness**: Rose, Geranium , Vetiver
- **Oils for relaxation and calm**: Lavender, camomile, benzoin
- **Oils for concentration**: Vetiver, Rosemary, basil

**Finger Paints**

Pair up your dough with matching oils for those extra special tots!

For these we use small plastic bottles or tubs, but you could use glass jars at a push as long as mum watched them carefully. How many you can make obviously depends on the size of the container!

- 2 cups cold water
- 1 heaped tbs cornflour (Corn starch)
- Food colouring
- Essential oils

Place the cornflower into a saucepan and carefully add the cold water.

Stir till all the lumps have gone.

Turn the heat on the burner and cook the mixture until it thickens.

Let it cool then pour into the bottles.

Add colouring and one drop of essential oil to each. Stir well with the wrong end of a teaspoon.

## Scented Pencils
This is very en vogue with aromatherapists at the moment. It is genius. I love it!

Buy unvarnished pencils and wipe oil along the edge with a cotton bud.

Love it…and again you can get therapeutic with your gift.

## Room Plaques
These are exactly the same idea as the pendants, but on a larger scale. You could try doing larger plaques saying "Love", "Sleep", "Gratitude" or even a child's name. These are great because all you need to do then in give then a couple of small phials of oils to top up the fragrance and their associated benefits

Here are a couple of ideas:

### Concentration
To fill a 1ml vial

- Vetiver - *(Vetiveria zizanoides)* x 3
- Rosemary (*Rosmarinus offinalis*) x 6
- Sweet Basil - (*Ocimum basilicum*) x 6
- Lemon *(Citrus limonum)* x 4

### Sleepy Time
- Lavender - (*Lavandula angustifolia*) x 10
- Camomile Roman (*Anthemis nobilis*) x 5
- Frankincense - (*Boswellia carterii*) x 5

### Happier Days
We all have days where the universe conspires against us. Being 6, is no different! Playground battles, sibling sulks and failed spelling tests can't compete with the happiness of this blend. They'll soon be smiling again.

- Bergamot - (*Citrus bergamia*) x 8
- Mandarin - (*Citrus reticulata*) x 6
- Benzoin - (*Styrax benzoin*) x 5

### Zap that Bug

Without getting too "clinical trial" on you, there is mountains of evidence of how simple essential oil vapours can overcome airborne pathogens. If you want to wipe out a nasty germ, use this blend.

- Tea Tree (*Maleleuca alternifolia*) x 6
- Clove (*Syzygium aromaticum*) x 6
- Oregano (*Origanum vulgare*) x 2
- Lemon (*Citrus limonum*) x 2

## The Garden

Dad and grandad then, because let's be honest, scented drawer liners isn't really going to cut it, is it?

Don't forget you can team these with bath salts for bad backs and hand creams too. Be creative, they don't have to be gardeners...

## Sunburn lotion

Make standard <u>body lotion</u> mix (see the beauty counter section)

- Cardamom (*Eletaria cardomum*) x 1
- Peppermint (*Mentha piperita*) x 1
- Spikenard (*Nardostachys jatamansi*) x 2
- Lavender - (*Lavandula angustifolia*) x 2

## Mosquito repellent

Make this as a lotion, a hand cream, an evaporator...whatever you think.

- 100ml base
- Citronella (*Cymbopgon nardus*) x 2
- Catnip (*Nepeta cataria*) x 2
- Vetiver - (*Vetiveria zizanoides*) x 1

## Insect Repellent Garden Twine

Now we girls won't get this, but I promise you lads do. It is worth making it just to watch how funny they are when they realise what it is.

Use it to tie up beans, peas etc. and the oils in twine keep away unwanted visitors. Campers, fishermen, gardeners...they all love this one.

- Use natural twine and get an old tin coffee canister.
- Paint or decorate your tin to taste...
- Peirce a hole in the top of the can to feed the string through.
- Now pour your essential oils into the tin and make sure that the string thoroughly soaks them up.
- It will continue to travel up the string for ages after you have done it.
- You are going to have to make about 10ml of oil for a whole spool of twin, so use 3 ml of each oil.
- Use a piece of sticky tape to secure the end of the string in place and keep the oil vapour trapped within.

**Insect Repellent Plant Markers**

Create lovely clay markers for the herb garden, following the same instructions as for the room plaques, but this time shape into little signposts and write names on and use the same catnip/vetiver mix as above.

# Conclusion

Goodness, the world has become such an easy shopping mall! When I qualified you could spend years trying to find out how to make a product. As for getting the ingredients, well it was legal minefield requiring all manner of documentation and licenses. Not any more, you got it easy, peasy guys.

It's great too, because there are so many different ways to use essential oils and we just tend not to talk about them in therapy. I would be the first to admit I am lazy with these things. Previously it was a pot of cream all the way, so it has been great fun widening my horizons a little bit.

Don't let's go too far the other way though. Let's be really careful about being nonchalant about these gifts we create. Just because it is *just* a bottle of ink or a bath bomb, doesn't mean it hasn't any properties. At every cross roads think about what the oils will do, how they will coax the physiology of the body, spark the mind or ease the spirit; respect the medicine of the plant...*and then* enjoy its fragrance.

I want to end this book in the same place I started it, with Jessie J....

*It's not about the money money, money, we wanna make the world dance. Forget about the price tag.*

Remember that. Happiness is in your hands. Use liberally...rinse and repeat!!!

Enjoy your creating and have a wonderful holiday season. As ever thanks so much for giving me a couple of hours of your time and please, if you have a second to spare, leave me a review. Lots of love, speak soon, Liz xxx

## About the Author

Elizabeth Ashley qualified as an aromatherapist in 1993, and then passed her Advanced Aromatherapy Diploma in 1994. She has been practicing aromatherapy for almost 22 years.

In 1999, she fell into a whole new career in the aggressive commercial sector of recruitment consultancy. There she discovered her father's second hand car salesman genes had passed along and found she had quite a gift of the gab! More than that, she discovered she could sell...and then some.

In 2008, Elizabeth fell ill during pregnancy with a blood clot in her lungs. The pulmonary embolism prevented her from working and she started to write. Very quickly she gained her first contract as a ghost writer...a recipe book for cheese cakes!

In 2010 she was published professionally for her work on Galbanum - (Ferula Galbaniflua) oil in the Aromatherapy Thymes, journal of the International Federation of Aromatherapists, and on TubeRose - (Rosa damascena) oil by the New Zealand Register of Holistic Therapist.

In 2011 she was seconded on a consultative basis to Walsall Independent Treatment Centre, designed to be a rainbow bridge between traditional and complementary medicines. There she became aware of the rumblings of change in healthcare. Her book Sales Strategies for Gentle Souls explains the connotations of this.

Many of her books are aimed at helping qualified aromatherapists to expand their healing repertoire and build their businesses. She also writes for people who have an interest in essential oils and want to learn how to heal. Her in depth essential oil profiles chart the healing properties of plants from the most arcane depths of historic folklore up to the scientific lab trials of today.

In 2014 she ranks in the top 50 contract writers on the freelancer marketplace Elance.com. She is the ghost writer of seven number one Amazon best sellers in the natural healing category. She lives in Shropshire with her husband and youngest son, kept company by their cat, the budgie and many shoals of tropical fish! Her elder son and daughter attend University and make her prouder than anything ever could.

Elizabeth Ashley is possibly one of the most published aromatherapy writers you have never heard of! By 2015, all of that will have changed. Elizabeth Ashley is The Secret Healer.

☐

## Other Books by the Author

Why not check out my reviews?

### In The Beauty Tips Range

50 Easy Essential Oil Recipes for Skin Care Products for Dry Skin - Make Your Own Anti-Aging Moisturizers & Night Creams

Professional Aromatherapy Skin Care Tips and Beauty Secrets

### The Secret Healer Oils Profiles:

Some of the oils we have covered in this book will be familiar, but possibly not all. You may find some of the oils profiles deepen your knowledge and fascination for the art of aromatherapy.

Vetiver - (Vetiveria zizanoides): the Oil of Tranquillity

Monarda: A Native American Medicine

Holy Basil: An Ayurvedic Medicine

Rose - (Rosa damascena): Goddess Medicine; A Timeless Elixir

Sweet Sweet Basil - (Ocimum basilicum)– The Oil of Empowerment

### The Secret Healing Manuals:

Book 1 - The Complete Guide to Clinical Aromatherapy & Essential Oils for the Physical Body

Download for FREE

Book 2 Essential Oils for Mind Body Spirit

The Holistic Medicine of Clinical Aromatherapy

Book 3 The Essential Oil Liver Cleanse

The Professional Aromatherapist's Liver Detox

Book 4 The Professional Stress Solution

Essential Oils and Holistic Health Stress Management Techniques for The Professional Aromatherapist

Book 5 The Aromatherapy Eczema Treatment

Healing Eczema, Itchy Skin Rashes and Atopic Dermatitis with Essential Oils and Holistic Medicine

Book 6 The Aromatherapy Bronchitis Treatment

Support the Respiratory System with Essential Oils and Holistic Medicine for COPD, Emphysema, Acute and Chronic Bronchitis Symptoms

Sales Strategies for Gentle Souls; Targeted Sales Training for Professional Aromatherapists

☐

# Disclaimer
by SEQ Legal

(1)     Introduction

This disclaimer governs the use of this book. [By using this book, you accept this disclaimer in full. / We will ask you to agree to this disclaimer before you can access the book.]


(2)     Credit

This disclaimer was created using an SEQ Legal template.


(3)     No advice

The book contains information about aromatherapy and the use of essential oils. The information is not advice, and should not be treated as such.


[You must not rely on the information in the book as an alternative to qualified medical advice from a health professional. advice from an appropriately qualified professional. If you have any specific questions about any medical matter you should consult an appropriately qualified professional.]

[If you think you may be suffering from any medical condition you should seek immediate medical attention. You should never delay seeking medical advice, disregard medical advice, or discontinue medical treatment because of information in the book.]

(4)     No representations or warranties

To the maximum extent permitted by applicable law and subject to section 6 below, we exclude all representations, warranties, undertakings and guarantees relating to the book.

Without prejudice to the generality of the foregoing paragraph, we do not represent, warrant, undertake or guarantee:

that the information in the book is correct, accurate, complete or non-misleading;

that the use of the guidance in the book will lead to any particular outcome or result; or in particular, that by using the guidance in the book you will heal disease or work in any way as a cure for illness.

(5)     Limitations and exclusions of liability

The limitations and exclusions of liability set out in this section and elsewhere in this disclaimer: are subject to section 6 below; and govern all liabilities arising under the disclaimer or in relation to the book, including liabilities arising in contract, in tort (including negligence) and for breach of statutory duty.

We will not be liable to you in respect of any losses arising out of any event or events beyond our reasonable control.

We will not be liable to you in respect of any business losses, including without limitation loss of or damage to profits, income, revenue, use, production, anticipated savings, business, contracts, commercial opportunities or goodwill.

We will not be liable to you in respect of any loss or corruption of any data, database or software.

We will not be liable to you in respect of any special, indirect or consequential loss or damage.

(6)   Exceptions

Nothing in this disclaimer shall: limit or exclude our liability for death or personal injury resulting from negligence; limit or exclude our liability for fraud or fraudulent misrepresentation; limit any of our liabilities in any way that is not permitted under applicable law; or exclude any of our liabilities that may not be excluded under applicable law.

(7)     Severability

If a section of this disclaimer is determined by any court or other competent authority to be unlawful and/or unenforceable, the other sections of this disclaimer continue in effect.

If any unlawful and/or unenforceable section would be lawful or enforceable if part of it were deleted, that part will be deemed to be deleted, and the rest of the section will continue in effect.

(8)     Law and jurisdiction

This disclaimer will be governed by and construed in accordance with English law, and any disputes relating to this disclaimer will be subject to the exclusive jurisdiction of the courts of England and Wales.

(9)     Our details

In this disclaimer, "we" means (and "us" and "our" refer to) [Build Your Own Reality)] of [Sy8 1LQ].